High Blood Pressure

William Campbell Douglass, MD

Rhino Publishing, S.A.

High Blood Pressure

ISBN 9962-636-60-4

Cover illustration by
Alex Manyoma (alex@3dcity.com)

Please, visit Rhino's website for other publications from
Dr. William Campbell Douglass
www.rhinopublish.com

Dr. Douglass' "Real Health" alternative medical
newsletter is available at www.realhealthnews.com

RHINO PUBLISHING, S.A.
World Trade Center
Panama, Republic of Panama
Voicemail/Fax
International: + 416-352-5126
North America: 888-317-6767

Other Books by
William Campbell Douglass, MD

- *Add 10 Years To Your Life*
- *Aids And Biological Warfare*
- *Bad Medicine*
- *Color Me Healthy*
- *Dangerous Legal Drugs: The Poisons In Your Medicine Chest*
- *Dr. Douglass Complete Guide To Better Vision*
- *Eat Your Cholesterol! -- Meat, Milk, And Butter -- And Live Longer*
- *Grandma Bell's A To Z Guide To Healing*
- *Hormone Replacement Therapies: Astonishing Results For Men And Women.*
- *Hydrogen Peroxide - Medical Miracle*
- *Into The Light - Tomorrow's Medicine Today*
- *Lethal Injections - Why Immunizations Don't Work*
- *Painful Dilemma -- Patients In Pain -- People In Prison*
- *Prostate Problems: Safe, Simple Effective Relief*
- *St. Petersburg Nights*
- *Stop Aging Or Slow The Process: Exercise With Oxygen Therapy*
- *The Eagle's Feather*
- *The Joy Of Mature Sex And How To Be A Better Lover...*
- *The Smoker's Paradox: The Health Benefits Of Tobacco*

Introduction:

We recently published in REAL HEALTH an article on high blood pressure and the current misconceptions about it both among the public and the doctors. It drew considerable attention. Because of the interest in the problem, and the misconceptions extant, we are offering to you a chapter from my upcoming book on cardiovascular disease: _THE POLITICALLY INCORRECT HEALTHY HEART BOOK_. We are offering this chapter now because, being over worked and over paid, I don't know when I will finish the book.

HYPERTENSION
-- WHAT IS IT?

I am not <u>always</u> politically-incorrect and, in the case of the treatment of hypertension, I have come to the middle of the road -- a dangerous place to be. I am not convinced that the prolonged treatment of <u>moderate</u> hypertension with drugs will prolong life. However, with severe hypertension the doctor has to treat with drugs, whether he really believes in them or not. The patient can visualize his head exploding from a hemorrhage -- and he may be right; it could happen. I am not convinced, however, that prolonged treatment of even these severe cases prolongs the life of the patient, but the treatment is based on that assumption -- and we have nothing else to offer in these, fortunately, rare cases.

The bad news is, there is no good news as far as alternative therapies for hypertension are concerned. By that I mean there is no <u>new</u> good news. Chelation therapy has a good record for consistently lowering the pressure and there are other helpful modalities which I will iterate subsequently. But there have been no "breakthroughs" -- in drug or natural therapies.

Blood pressure is measured as two values. <u>Systolic</u>, the first, or top, number, is the pressure inside arteries when the heart beats, that is, squeezes down to pump the blood into that vast arterial network coursing to the outer reaches of your body.

Diastolic, the last number, is the pressure between beats when the heart is at rest. Ideal blood pressure is 120 over 80, or lower. High blood pressure is above 140 over 90. (There is some quibble in this.)

An elevated blood pressure, "hypertension," has always been a mystery. It has been blamed on the kidneys (renin), environmental pollution, "stress," arteriosclerosis, a rigid personality, the thyroid, anger, the adrenal medulla, the adrenal cortex, obesity, excessive alcohol consumption, erythropoietin, sleep apnea, insulin, sodium chloride (salt), hormones, a stiffening of the arteries or a combination of some of the above. Because of the possibility of a combination of causes, which can vary with the patient, the determination of an exact causation in a particular case is usually not feasible.

Hypertension is designated as primary, essential (which makes no sense to me) or idiopathic, which simply means "We don't know." Actually, all of these terms mean we don't know. While some cases of hypertension have a distinct etiology, pheochromocytoma for example, the large majority do not have a known cause and we will limit our discussion to this group. If you have high blood pressure -- hypertension -- you are probably in this cohort of many millions of Americans with "essential hypertension," "idiopathic hypertension," or "primary" hypertension," -- take your pick; they're all the same.

CYSTOLIC OR DIASTOLIC OR BOTH?

We were taught in medical school at the mid-century that the systolic (upper) pressure wasn't as important as the diastolic (lower) pressure. The assumption was that the constant extra pressure, caused by the elevated diastolic number, was the reason it was more important than an elevated systolic (upper) number. The constant additional pressure would, over the long term, be more destructive than the temporary additional pressure of the systolic phase.

"Millions of Americans don't have their high blood pressure under control, and one reason is that some doctors still believe an old myth that systolic pressure - the top number in your reading - isn't really important, health officials said..." reports Lauran Neergaard of the Associated Press. "Systolic hypertension is a major under emphasized threat, particularly for older people, even if their diastolic pressure, the bottom number, is perfectly normal," says a National Institutes of Health advisory to physicians.

"Unfortunately, many physicians have not yet ... become aggressive in treating such patients," said Dr. Daniel Levy, director of the National Heart, Lung and Blood Institute's Framingham Heart Study and co-author of the advisory. Maybe it's unfortunate and maybe it isn't.

Being ever suspicious about the continuing commercialization of American medicine, I am not ready to agree with this "new discovery" that isolated systolic hypertension in the elderly needs pharmacologic treatment. This will open up a gigantic market of previously undetected disease. It always seemed to me that a certain amount of stiffening can be expected in the arteries as one ages. This would increase the systolic (upper number) pressure due to the blood pushing against a more resistant arterial wall. I don't know if physiologists have proven this but it's my interpretation of the matter. Is it a good idea to drive down the systolic pressure in a resistant artery? I don't know, but we need to find out before jumping in to this one. There is a tremendous risk of doing more harm than good here.

An estimated 50 million Americans have high blood pressure, often called the "silent killer" <u>because it may not cause symptoms until the patient has suffered serious damage to the arterial system</u>. It raises the risk of heart attacks, strokes, congestive heart failure, kidney damage, dementia and even blindness. That's a laundry list of horrors you want to avoid and so drug treatment should be an easy sell to the public.

According to the NIH advisory, only a quarter of hypertensives are "adequately controlled." This, they say, is primarily due to inadequate control of systolic pressure. There is a massive campaign going on to educate the public to the

NEW PARADIGM: "Early detection means early treatment and cure" -- just like with the American Cancer Society and the war on breast cancer. And like the war on breast cancer, it may turn out to just as disappointing. Early drug treatment <u>may not work at all</u> to reduce the mortality rate. It needs to be tried, however, <u>IF</u> they can find drugs that won't do more harm than good.

In one study, patients treated for "isolated systolic hypertension" (upper reading high, lower reading normal) cut their risk of heart failure by more than 50 percent and the risk of stroke and heart attacks by a third. "That's a pretty dramatic lowering of risk," Levy said.

I don't know how you could prove that but I hope it's true.

Another example of therapeutic success in the Neergaard report: A pressure is 160 over 100, and a first attempt at medication drops it to 148 over 86. Doctors assume the bottom number is low enough to stop treatment, but ``you need to press on until you get the systolic to less than 140,'' one of the research doctors said. I'm not sure that "pressing on" is a good idea in these patients, who are usually elderly. Some studies have indicated that treatment to lower "isolated systolic hypertension" increases mortality.

Hypertension treatment is the same regardless of whether the problem is systolic or diastolic or both. But what if they have different mechanisms? Then you will need two drugs, which greatly increases your potential for serious side effects. Diet, exercise, potassium supplements chelation therapy and <u>practically anything but drugs</u> is the way to go in my opinion. We'll discuss alternatives below.

Ref: Associated Press, 5/4/00, Lauran Neergaard

HYDROPHILIA AND HYPERTENSION

About five years ago, I first became aware of a peculiar new fad (At least I thought it was peculiar). Everybody seemed to be gorging on water from plastic bottles. People (more women, it seems) always seemed to have the bottle at the ready, in case of a dehydration attack, I suppose. They slug H2O down the old gullet just about anywhere, under most any circumstance – in the middle of giving a lecture, sitting on the sidewalk, at funerals or other festivities – they drink it as though the Sahara desert was only a bottle-throw away. Even the commander of forces in Afghanistan was seen on world television standing at the lectern sucking on a water bottle.

The maximum in hydro chic is to carry your water in a holster so as to affect a quick draw, to avoid the aforementioned general pruning of your skin, and the shrinking of your innards -- you don't want a shrunken liver, do you? "Your Body Cries Out for Water!" (over sold idea, in my opinion)

There is a simple mechanism that will tell you when you need water. It's called thirst. But, what if you are drinking <u>too much</u> water? How would you know it? Your answer – especially if you are a confirmed hydrophiliac – is that "you can't drink too much water."

Now there is solid scientific evidence that you <u>can</u> drink too much water, especially if you are over 60 or have hypertension or heart disease. For reasons not understood, drinking water increases blood pressure profoundly in patients with autonomic failure <u>and substantially in older patients.</u> Don't worry about that "autonomic failure" business. The point I wish to make here is that <u>healthy elderly people</u>, not to speak of the unhealthy ones, can have <u>a considerable rise in blood pressure</u> by drinking too much water. With a heavy water load, systolic blood pressure increased by 11 mm Hg in elderly <u>but not in young controls.</u>

The authors concluded that heavy imbibition of water raises plasma norepinephrine ("speed") as much as caffeine and nicotine!

Action to take:

(1) If you have a blood pressure problem, and are on medication, <u>don't tank up on fluids before your doctor visit.</u> He may think you need a higher dose of medicine, where all you really needed was a trip to the bathroom.

(2) Don't force yourself to drink water if you are not thirsty (I never touch the stuff.), or unless a doctor has advised "forcing fluids" for a medical reason. I don't mean to imply that I do not take in any water. Water is in practically everything you eat and certainly everything you drink – even your 100-proof Old Granddad bourbon is half water. So is milk, so is a commercial chicken.

Ref: Circulation, Feb. 8, 2000

HEREDITY AND HYPERTENSION

Before you ask, yes, there are hereditary factors but these have not been clearly defined. If you have close relatives -- mother, father, siblings -- with hypertension, you may also contract this condition, but not necessarily.

ATHEROSCLEROSIS AND HYPERTENSION

"Accelerated atherosclerosis is an invariable companion of hypertension," states Dr. Gordon H. Williams in Harrison's Textbook of Medicine. There has been enough research in this age of hypertension to establish that unequivocal opinion, I suppose. However, his extrapolation that follows will lead to more confusion: "Thus, it is not surprising that independent risk factors associated with the development of atherosclerosis, such as an elevated serum cholesterol....enhance the effect of hypertension on mortality rate."

<u>There is no good evidence that an elevated serum cholesterol per se causes atherosclerosis</u>. This important subject, the role of cholesterol in your health, is discussed in Chapter....

As for hardening of the arteries causing hypertension, it follows, from a physiological standpoint, that arteries that are inflexible will cause an elevated pressure.

HYPERTENSION AND WEIGHT REDUCTION

The debate on how best to lose weight goes on interminably. The truth of the matter is that there are many ways to lose weight, some of them rational and safe and some not. Although they are diametrically opposed to each other, the Adkins diet and the Ornish barn feed diet will both work. The Adkins diet is rational and scientifically-based whereas the Ornish diet is not.

Yes, I know he has Harvard on his side but that does not necessarily mean that his diet recommendations are not political and financially motivated --just like a lot of other stuff that comes out of Harvard. Ornish likes to brag about his White House connections (a least he did under the Clintonistas) but I don't consider that exactly a recommendation in his favor either.

Douglas Lisle, PH.D and Alan Goldhammer, D.C. (chiropractor) have reproduced a graph that, if accurate, tells reams about the diet hoopla. Also, it reveals a lot about the biases of the people who put the graph together.

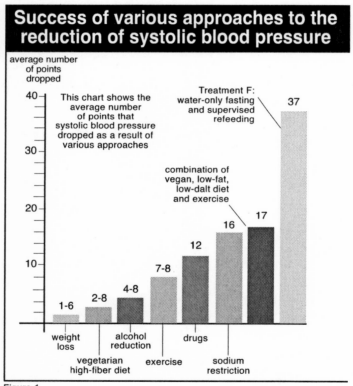

Success of various approaches to the reduction of systolic blood pressure

average number of points dropped

This chart shows the average number of points that systolic blood pressure dropped as a result of various approaches

Treatment F: water-only fasting and supervised refeeding

combination of vegan, low-fat, low-dalt diet and exercise

40 — 37

30 —

20 — 17

16

12

10 — 7-8

4-8

2-8

1-6

weight loss | alcohol reduction | drugs
vegetarian high-fiber diet | exercise | sodium restriction

Figure 1

Note that this study concerns itself with only one of the parameters of the cardiovascular problem, blood pressure, and that is a logical approach. Keep it simple and you are more likely to come up with results that are meaningful.

Weight loss alone; a vegetarian, high-fiber diet and alcohol reduction alone revealed poor-to-negligible blood pressure reduction. The next four dietary and life-style changes -- exercise, drugs, sodium restriction and the Ornish/ MacDougal type of vegan food only, low-fat, low-salt and exercise, were impressive.

But is the dark blue column, with the 17 mm Hg on top of it, really impressive? If you alter four parameters -- low fat, vegan-only food, exercise and low salt intake -- <u>you then get only one mm Hg improvement over simply restricting salt intake.</u>

Aren't you just baptizing broccoli here? Aren't you missing out on some great chateaubriand, veal scaloppini and chicken soup? What is the point of this? Do you really want to risk a shortened life, leukemia or a stroke (or all of the above) for the privilege of eating the equivalent of <u>vegetarian cat food</u> for the rest of your life.

(Parenthetically, and that's why this is in parentheses, if you have a cat, feed it nothing but raw chicken liver once a day and it will live a disease-free life -- and probably out live you.)

Also note that if you remove the salt restriction and the exercise factors, the tall dark blue column, proudly proclaiming its superiority in hypertension control, will wilt down to the lower classes, i.e., down there with vegan/high fiber (the dark brown column) -- which is where it belongs.

And now the prejudice I mentioned above that is clearly revealed in this graph.

The *Rabbit/Rhinoceros Food for the Masses* crowd are so prejudiced against the believers in a normal, omniverous diet for humans and are so convinced that they are right -- and all past nutrition research and historical nutritional information is wrong -- that they will not reveal the results of a diet that drastically restricts sugar, starch and high-sugar containing fruits and vegetables, but includes meat and the fat of meat.

I am referring, of course, to the recommended diets of pioneers like Weston Price, George Mann, the Doctors Pinckney and Robert Adkins. If you did a study on the effect on blood pressure of a strict Adkins diet, I suspect that the result on blood pressure would be as good as any of these, including the low-salt diet. Why didn't they include this diet regimen in their study since they know that millions of people are doing it with excellent effect on their health?

As for the "water-only diet" (big red there, with the 37 on top), <u>starvation will work every time</u>. After the practitioner has starved you to his satisfaction, he slides you into a vegan diet -- semi starvation -- and that is where you, presumably, will stay for the rest of your miserable vegan life. <u>Any diet that lowers your blood pressure by 37 mm Hg is dangerous</u>. And I recommend that you not attempt it unless you are under the supervision of a <u>qualified MD</u>, not some clown practicing medicine with a Ph. D, or with a pseudo medical degree, or with his driver's license.

In summary, weight reduction is considered by most practitioners of medicine -- both allo-pathic and non-drug advocates -- to be primary in control of blood pressure. Although it is not a cure-all, it is important and should be the first line of offense against this stubborn advisory.

Let's look at another study. (Can you take one more?)

Anastasia Georgiades, Ph.D., of the department of psychiatry and behavioral science at Duke University Medical Center in Durham, has done a study measuring the effect on blood pressure of weight reduction and exercise as a combination treatment. Dr. Georgiades is a psychologist, or I assume she is. (If you work in the department of psychiatry and you have a Ph.D., doesn't that make you a psychologist?)

Individuals in the exercise/weight loss group in this study had an average decrease in systolic pressure of 8 points. That's pretty fair and comparable to what the graph shown above can be done with <u>exercise alone</u>.

In the exercise-only group, the average systolic reading dropped by 3.5 points. This is only half the decrease in the exercise component of the graph illustrated above and reveals the disparity in results found in multi factorial studies.

"The research placed particular emphasis on the importance of reducing blood pressure at times of increased mental stress," reported Medscape Wire.

"Our results show that exercise and weight loss helped to keep blood pressure lower even when individuals were under mental stress," says Georgiades. "Like high blood pressure itself," she continued, "an exaggerated cardiovascular response to mental stress is an additional risk factor for heart disease."

<u>Many studies have shown that "stress" has little or nothing to do with elevated blood pressure</u>. I thought we had put that old shrink's fairy tale to rest but here it is again from the department of psychiatry of a major university.

"Exercise and weight management programs also resulted in health benefits such as a lower heart rate, more efficient pumping of the heart, greater dilation of blood vessels and a higher overall level of fitness, according to the study," said the reporter from Medscape Wire. I wonder how they measured all these wonderful improvements and if the data will be in their published version of the study.

If they ran an exercise-only group, why didn't they run a weight-reduction-only group as well?

Ref: MedscapeWire, August 18, 2000

Hypertension, 8/00

BLOOD PRESSURE AND SUNLIGHT

Theresa Tamkins of Reuters news service reported:

"....lack of exposure to ultraviolet light may actually contribute to the rise in blood pressure in higher latitudes, according to a new theory from an Alabama researcher. And the theory may explain why blacks in the U.S. and Europe have a greater risk of high blood pressure than whites in those countries or blacks who live in Africa."

Well, it is not a "new theory." I first reported on this blood pressure/light connection <u>ten years ago</u> in my book, *Into the Light,* and in my medical newsletter. Anyway, the farther one gets from the equator, going either up or down, the more likely you are to find high blood pressure.

I always liked the theory about blacks having less hypertension in Africa because the sun is more intense there. But, recent investigations in Uganda reveal that hypertension is <u>skyrocketing</u> in African countries, especially in the cities. So we are "back to square zero," as my African friends like to put it. We can assume that hypertension in Uganda is due primarily to years of poor nutrition, just like everywhere else. Not that lack of ultraviolet light isn't a factor in hypertension with blacks as well a whites -- more blacks will have hypertension in Jamaica, New York than in Jamaica, Greater Antilles.

The further one gets from the equator, the less ultraviolet Light and the less vitamin D that is synthesized in the skin. This phenomenon is not only pigment-related but age-related. As the skin ages, it becomes less efficient in absorbing ultraviolet and, consequently, less vitamin D is manufactured. This is a strong reason for the family not to limit cod liver oil consumption to the kids. It should be a family affair. Adults should take four capsules twice a day; kids -- two capsules twice daily.

Cod liver oil consumption is particularly important in people with dark skin. This is not a racial thing. Whether you are from India, Cambodia (where people also have black skin) or Tanzania, hypertension is more likely to be a problem as these diverse racial types move away from the sun, i.e., to the far north. People with very dark skin require six times the amount of ultraviolet B light to produce the same amount of vitamin D found in people of lighter skin color.

A refined method of treatment with sunlight is "photoluminescence," the treatment of a small amount of the patient's blood with ultraviolet light, which is then reinjected into the patient. This may have a profound effect on the blood pressure in a hypertensive patient. American research in this promising field has been essentially nil since the 1940s. And hypertension per se I don't believe has ever been studied, using UV light therapy, in this country. A lowering of pressure has been noted incidental to the treatment of other conditions.

However the Russians have studied the treatment of hypertension with UV light and have had impressive results. Dr. Igor Dutkevich, with whom I worked at Hospital 15 in St. Petersburg, Russia, has reported promising results as has the Azerbaijan Republican Hospital in Baku. Their method would seem to be over treatment to me, but it is hard to argue with good results. The patients received five to ten treatments every other day -- about five times what I would consider a safe maximum. Many patients had a lowering of the pressure of 30 percent and the use of drugs was drastically reduced.

This research needs to be repeated in this country but it will not happen in my lifetime.

"There are multiple factors that contribute to blood pressure control," said Dr. Paul Velletri, the hypertension group leader at the National Heart, Lung, and Blood Institute in Bethesda, Maryland... "I don't think it's likely that it would be a sole cause for hypertension for most people," Velletri said to reporter, Theresa Tamkins of Reuters.

I agree with Dr. Valletri. Hypertension is a multifactorial disease. However, we can now add lack of sunlight (ultraviolet) to the hypertension equation -- call it "photopenia." (I like to create neologisms.)

Ref: Hypertension, 1997;30:150-156

HIGH BLOOD PRESSURE AND OSTEOPOROSIS

Women with high blood pressure face an increased risk of developing the brittle bone disease, osteoporosis, according to a recent report.

The research, on more than 3,600 women, confirms what doctors have long suspected.

Researchers found that elderly women with high blood pressure suffered bone thinning at a rate nearly twice that experienced by other women, The Lancet reports. This is not surprising as it is known that high blood pressure causes loss of calcium in the body and loss of bone strength. But the <u>reason</u> for this effect is not known. The head researcher in this report wants to blame it on salt, but I have my doubts.

Dr Francesco Cappuccio, of St George's Hospital, London, UK, studied women in Baltimore, Minneapolis, Portland and Pittsburgh. Cappuccio says there is evidence suggesting that cutting salt consumption can help stem the loss of calcium. He concludes: "Decreased salt intake should lessen the risk of osteoporosis and hip fractures in elderly people and also have a blood pressure lowering effect."

<u>Salt does not cause hypertension</u> in most people; therefore reducing salt intake will not lower blood pressure, except in susceptible peo-

ple. A prori, reducing salt is not a cure-all or pre-ventive for osteoporosis. Only fifty percent of people are salt-sensitive -- some say much less. Dr. Cappucchio needs to start over and select salt-sensitive people for his research before jump-ing to conclusions about salt restriction for everybody with hypertension.

HYPERTENSION – THE SEARCH FOR A CURE

Combining weight loss and exercise lowers blood pressure more effectively than exercise alone, according to an article in the Archives of Internal Medicine. Everyone gets the same advice from their doctor: Exercise and eat a "healthy diet." The problem is most doctors don't know what a healthy diet is – they have been badly mislead by the American Heart Association, the American Dietetic Association and all the rest of the cabala that worships the fearsome Janus of fat/cholesterol.

The study of 133 overweight men and women with untreated hypertension found that about an hour of exercise three to four times a week for six months reduced blood pressure and weight loss lowered it more.

"These findings provide further evidence for the effectiveness of non-pharmacological approaches to treating hypertension," said Dr. James Blumenthal of Duke University Medical Center, the senior researcher in the Duke study.

I don't think the study provides any evidence at all.

Members of the weight loss and exercise group lowered their systolic blood pressure, the top number, by an average of 7 points. Let's say your systolic pressure is 160. A reduction of seven points is well within the range of the placebo effect, about four percent. If the appearance of a man in a white coat, the doctor, can cause a 20 percent rise in pressure, it is not surprising that all this attention by doctor and staff should lower the pressure at least a little.

I have a lady friend of 40 years who has a pressure around 180/90. She has had this high reading for at least 20 years. Bobbie, a beautiful redhead, is five-foot-two-inches tall, weighs about 90 pounds, never smoked and doesn't exercise. She feels fine and refuses BP medication. They make her so ill that she knows if she takes them they will kill her. She is 60 and remains asymptomatic. Is she sitting on a time bomb or disproving the experts? When she is 80, and has lived her four score, I'll check her out. (I'll only be 94.)

So what do we know about hypertension after 75 years of studying it? We can prevent it in most cases of "essential" hypertension, if the patient is willing to live within certain constraints. Of course, you can't prove you prevented something if it doesn't happen. That's the curse that goes with the practice of preventive medicine: If you prevent it, you get no credit; if they get it, you're responsible for not preventing it. That's why it is better to write about medicine than to practice it.

Severe hypertension may not respond to diet/exercise/weight loss and drugs may have to be resorted to in combination with the non-drug methods described herein. This is where I land in the middle of the road, mentioned at the beginning of this chapter. However, drugs should be a last resort and there should be an on-going effort to reduce the dosage of drugs and total elimination when possible. They are clearly a two-edge sword.

Ref: Archives of Internal Medicine, 7/10/00

####

TREATING HYPERTENSION WITH CHEMICALS

A national survey reveals that nearly 19 million Americans are at risk <u>from their own medications</u>.

A national anti hypertensive medication survey was released on November 10, 1999, in a symposium sponsored by the Association of Black Cardiologists, Inc. (ABC) The study showed that <u>38 percent of patients stop their medication because of intolerable side effects</u>. The rate is probably higher than that because patients lie to the doctor so as not to hurt his feelings. This is another aspect of the "white coat syndrome." (Blood pressure tends to rise in the doctor's office and now we can add: The rate of prevarication rises in the doctor's office.) The study also illustrates how ineffective pharmaceuticals are in the treatment of hypertension.

With apparently no sense that he was admitting the major failure of conventional cardiovascular drug medicine, Dr. Frank James, President of the ABC, said, "This survey highlights the extent of the tolerability problem in hypertension, which is widespread among all patient populations, and underscores the need for the medical community to continue searching for pharmacological alternatives."

Well, the "medical community" doesn't search for pharmacological alternatives, Frank. The multi-billion-dollar drug industry does that and the doctor merely uses the improved version of "PressureGlow" without having the slightest idea how the drug was tested, or how many beagles they killed in testing, or how many <u>people</u> they killed for that matter.

And why should we be looking for "pharmacological alternatives"? Talk about begging the question – chemical, i.e., "pharmacological," treatment of high blood pressure is <u>a failure</u>. Why do doctors pretend a treatment works when it has become obvious that it doesn't? Cancer chemotherapy is another apt example of this Alice-in-Wonderland mentality: "Keep treating, even if it makes the patient sicker; something may turn up and, in the meantime, we have to do <u>something</u>."

"Surprisingly," Dr. James continues, "the survey also presents some new challenges in treating high blood pressure, because the findings show that elevated systolic blood pressure is not being controlled to the recommended levels." Dr. James could get to be known as the Alan Greenspan of Medicine if he keeps talking like that. What he is saying in his euphemistic doctor way is that <u>the drugs aren't working</u>. Frank, don't you get it? Why are you "surprised"? It's been obvious for <u>50 years</u> that drug therapy for hypertension is a <u>dead end</u>.

Blood pressure-lowering drugs include <u>diuretics</u> (Diueril) , to reduce fluid retention; <u>beta blockers</u>, which inhibit the sympathetic nervous system; <u>ACE</u> drugs, which inhibit the formation of blood vessel-narrowing enzymes; and <u>calcium channel blockers</u> that reduce oxygen utilization and interfere with the normal constriction and relaxation of coronary arteries. (We'll tell you more about this "wonder drug" below.)

I started pushing drugs for the "legitimate" drug industry – also called the "ethical" drug industry – in 1950. My big seller was "Maxitate," mannitol hexanitrate. The packaging was beautiful. The doctors fell for it and I was becoming a star with the company. However, I began to realize that, although the drug wasn't apparently hurting anybody, <u>it wasn't working</u>.

So I quit and went to medical school. We've been through many drugs since then – beta blockers, diuretics, ACE inhibitors, and the group that was touted to be the sure-fire answer to hypertension, the calcium channel blockers. We've passed a lot of water since I was a drug dealer -- and the drugs <u>still</u> don't work for hypertension.

The pharmaceutical approach does not attempt to address the basic issues of hypertension -- laziness and gluttony. Most "essential hypertension" is a <u>dietary problem</u> combined with <u>laziness</u>.

By gluttony I mean the unwillingness to eat less and to eat close to zero starch and sugar. We are a nation addicted to sugar; the number two addiction is starch and these are followed by cigarettes and alcohol. If you own a liquor store and an ice cream parlor, you will never be broke. Since free enterprise erupted in Russia, I noted, when living in St. Petersburg, that some of the mobsters (excuse me, I meant "businessmeni") have combined the two -- ice cream parlors that sell liquor. And so back to the subject....

Most doctors don't seem to consider that high blood pressure is not a disease per se. As with a fever, which is the body's reaction to an infection, hypertension may be the physiological response of the body to some internal threat. That "internal threat," more often than not, is too many biscuits, too much apple pie and too much diet Coke.

You can no more treat hypertension successfully with drugs alone than you can treat a septicemia with aspirin.

Diuretics, for example, such as the commonly prescribed hydrochlorothiazide (HCTZ), eliminate sodium along with fluid from your body, and so can cause an imbalance in the body's crucial sodium/potassium ratio. Calcium channel blockers, such as verapamil hydrochloride, upset the calcium/magnesium balance, and can cause tissue cells to lose their calcium. Beta blockers, such as propranolol, counter the normal effects of adrenal hormones on heart action. ACE, such as captopril, interrupt the normal hormonal functions of the kidneys and affect how they filter sodium and water.

The most commonly reported side effects were fatigue (22%), and dizziness (21%). Of patients treated with beta-blockers, the average percentage of patients having fatigue as a side effect is 34 percent.

• Of patients treated with diuretics, the average percentage of patients experiencing electrolyte imbalance as a side effect is 30 percent.

• Of patients treated with calcium channel blockers, the average percentage of patients having edema (excess fluid in the tissues) as a side effect is 26 percent.

- Of patients treated with ACE inhibitors, the average percentage of patients having cough as a side effect is 21 percent. Edema, fatigue and dizziness are bad enough. But when you experience cough as a side effect, any doctor cognizant of the side effects of drugs will be immediately concerned about the onset of <u>pulmonary fibrosis</u> -- a serious and non-reversible, drug-induced disease of the lungs.

Side effects are not the only problem. Seventy-five percent of treating physicians reported in the study that drug-drug interactions are a common problem with their patients. That means two or more drugs interacting and causing "adverse events." <u>Thirty-six percent of patients take three to five other medications</u>. So there is plenty of room for mischief here. <u>Forty-six percent</u> of patients take 2 to 3 other medications. As you may surmise, this is not an exact science we are dealing with.

In the study that Dr. James is reviewing here, there was a reported success rate of 65 percent. (This is probably falsely high as the White Coat Syndrome has to be factored in as well as the placebo effect, positive as well a negative -- see below.) Some studies have reported success rates of only 50 percent to as low as 30 percent. Now you are in the placebo-effect range. However, it is what I call a "negative placebo effect" -- "Since I started the drug I feel worse, therefore, I must be getting better."

A MUTT AMONG DOGS --
CALCIUM CHANNEL BLOCKERS

Thirty years ago, "calcium channel blockers" became the latest and the greatest family of drugs that were going to control hypertension, once and for all. By that time in my medical career, I was skeptical of the "latest and the greatest" drug cure in ANY field of medicine. In retrospect, my skepticism was justified.

An extensive study has shown that the Calcium Channel Blockers are no better than the older drugs for lowering pressure, the major difference is the price -- the CCBs are more expensive. But that is only the beginning of the indictment against the CCB drugs.

In a review of nine studies that included more than 27,000 people with high blood pressure, some interesting – and damning – statistics came to light concerning the CCBs.

According to a report in The Lancet, <u>patients taking CCBs were about 26% more likely to have a heart attack and 25% more likely to experience congestive heart failure</u> compared to patients taking ACE inhibitors, diuretics or beta-blockers. Also, their risk of any major cardiovascular event, including heart attack and heart failure, was 10% higher than with the older and cheaper drugs. Whew! Now that's an indictment with which even <u>a president</u> would have trouble.

Now don't dash to the bathroom and pour your CCBs in the toilet. You might cause an eco-logical disaster (What would it do to the frogs?) and besides, <u>you could drop dead</u>. I don't mean because you will be attacked by one of those coo coo carrot suckers or bear huggers, but because suddenly stopping these powerful drugs causes them to turn on you like a lover spurned. And it will attack exactly where you would expect it -- in your heart.

Dr. Marco Pahor, of Wake Forest University in Winston Salem, North Carolina, the lead author in the Lancet study said, rather diplomatically I thought, if patients are not taking blood pressure drugs that can also reduce the risk of heart dis-ease, "it is reasonable for them to ask why." (Reuters Health)

Not being much of a diplomat, I would have expressed it differently: "Why in hell are you tak-ing a drug that can kill you when it is no more effective for lowering blood pressure than cheaper drugs that are less likely to kill you?"

HIGH BLOOD PRESSURE AND NUTRITION

The most important nutrient in the nutritional treatment of hypertension is vitamin D. This nutrient is closely related to sunlight. If you don't get enough sunlight, your skin will not produce enougfh vitamin D and this will result in many health problems from rickets to high blood pressure. That does not mean that Vitamin D supplementation will cure hypertension. If it were only that simple.

Calcium is also important in the regulation of blood pressure. Its role in hypertension is also unclear and calcium alone will not cure hypertension.

Many herbals have been proven to have blood pressure lowering effects. In research done thus far, garlic seems most effective. Others with at least some effect are: Cayenne pepper, Fennel, Hawthorne, and Rosemary.

SUMMERIZING A SAD SITUATION

High blood pressure is a complex problem not easily treated. Even the best of doctors, conventional or holistic, may fail to control most patients' blood pressure on a permanent basis. Holistic methods (exercise, diet, chelation therapy, stress reduction, etc.) should be tried first.

As for the chemical approach, I am not convinced that the drugs are better than doing nothing. If the drug lowers your pressure, is it worth the cost, the cost in money and quality of life? Do drugs prolong life? That has not been proved and I doubt that they do. Studies have reported success rates of only 50 percent to as low as 30 percent. That is well within the placebo range, meaning that starch capsules would have worked as well.

There is a relationship between calcium metabolism, parathyroid hormone and high blood pressure, but the relationship is not clear at all. There are many complexities in treating this stubborn condition. Hypertension has been studied intensively for over 50 years -- during my entire career as a doctor. We learn more, about more and more, in the business of hypertension without making significant progress. At this point, the natural way -- weight reduction, an omniverous but low carbohydrate diet and exercise -- are the treatments of choice.

Ref: The Lancet December 9, 2000.
Merritt McKinney, Reuters Health
Association of Black Cardiologists press release,
11/15/99

####

SALT AND HYPERTENSION

I was taught that only ten percent of hypertensive patients are sensitive to salt. Now they say that 60 percent are sensitive. I don't know if that dramatic difference is a true change or whether I was misinformed in the first place -- or if the present figure is an exaggeration. Whatever the truth, the statistics indicate a lot of people are having their salt intake restricted, probably to their detriment.

Remember, salt and chloride are essential nutrients. Restricting their intake can lead to medical problems. Some years ago, a large and respected manufacturer of baby formula decided to limit the amount of chloride in the formula, based on the suggestion of some hotshot nutritionist/physiologist. It was a disaster and many babies died.

Babies, being similar to humans (at least before Wade vs Roe), had proved an important point: sodium, chloride and the combination, know as salt, are <u>essential nutrients</u> and so they are essential to good health. If you have serious hypertension, you may have to restrict your salt intake. However, make sure it is necessary in your case. Ask the doctor to do a salt challenge test.

Salt deprivation has been found to be a common cause of chronic fatigue syndrome. Recent studies indicate that chlorine, rather than the indicted sodium, may be the culprit -- look what happened to the babies in the above report. Even calcium may be a contributing factor.

I haven't reported on salt in over seven years. Since salt is one of your most important nutrients, an update is overdue. There has been a great deal of research since my 1994 report that essentially confirms my original hypothesis: Severe salt restriction in people – sick or well – is a dangerous practice and may be counterproductive.

The Kempner studies in 1944 and 1948 on treating hypertension with the "Rice diet" resulted in a paradigm shift in thinking about the role of salt and sodium in the diet. It became gospel that salt restriction was paramount in controlling hypertension. But, as so often happens in science, there was an over reaction. The studies were done on malignant hypertension, which is far removed from the average patient we see in practice with high blood pressure. In most practices, you are not likely to see more than a few cases of this magnitude of hypertension in your entire career, unless you work in a black community. And even in Kempner's study, only 50 percent of the patients showed any improvement at all on the rice diet. (Do you think you could live on a diet of rice, fruit and no salt?)

The Dahl studies of 1972 were even less realistic with a hodgepodge of variables that made the study useless. It never should have been published by the American Journal of Clinical Nutrition. The problem with all these studies is that the pesky, inattentive, uncomprehending and forgetful experimental animal – man – is difficult, if not impossible, to control.

There are additional problems. What else is he eating? Does he remember? (It's a wise man who knows his fodder.) Is he telling you what you want to hear? Is he sneaking salt? (People <u>love</u> salt, even people not afflicted with vegetarianism.) Even if the subjects are trying to cooperate, it is hard to quantitate salt intake. Practically every processed food bought contains added salt unless stated otherwise. Are the subjects required to read the labels? (Fat chance)

The frustration of uncertainty in a scientific pursuit in medicine eventually leads to "meta analysis." This is a technique of throwing all the relevant studies into a pot, mixing well and then analyzing various parameters, looking for a desired outcome. This method is highly suspect and will often lead to <u>compounding the errors</u> of the majority of the studies.

You're probably getting tired of this statistical stuff but it is important to know because now you'll be more skeptical of these soft studies which purport to be scientific. One more important criticism and then we will leave the over rated field of biostatistics.

There is the problem of <u>confounding factors</u> that can completely negate the best laid plans of mouse or man, and especially man. These factors can cause a reduction in blood pressure (or an elevation) not related at all to salt restriction such as: weight change, exercise, potassium intake, magnesium intake, alcohol (increase or decrease, depending on the patient), prescription and non-prescription drugs, a calamitous emotional event and others.

Lowering blood pressure by salt restriction is inconsistent and so unreliable. But there is a far worse criticism of salt restriction: Studies have shown that salt restriction may be linked to organ damage, especially kidney disease and left ventricular hypertrophy. Put simply: Restricting salt intake may be the worse thing you can do. If the heart and kidneys are damaged by hyponatremia (low blood sodium), you may make the hypertension worse.

After all this research, there is still no good way to check for sodium (salt) sensitivity. This is clearly needed as certain groups – blacks, the elderly and the obese – are those most likely to be salt sensitive. Some, but not drastic, salt restriction may improve control of hypertension in these patients.

The *Scottish Heart Study* of 11,000 Scottish men & women found no correlation between salt and blood pressure. The well known *Intersalt* study seemed to find clear evidence of a salt-hypertension correlation. But it turned out to be as porous as other studies that had proven "conclusively" that excess salt was responsible for hypertension. Furthermore, an eight-year follow-up of the *Scottish Heart Study* didn't change their opinion: "...(salt) had little predictive value for either coronary heart disease or all-cause mortality over an eight-year follow-up period." (Chrysant, *Progress in Cardiovascular Disease*, July/August, 1999)

Furthermore, even in those studies illustrating blood pressure reduction with salt restriction (the TOHP studies), the reduced pressure could not be sustained. Dr. George S. Chrysant, a leader in hypertensive research, commented on the TOHP research results: "weight loss was more effective in lowering blood pressure than sodium (salt) reduction.... and the effects of both interventions dissipated with time." He concluded: "....the high rates of recidivism ....despite intensive and expert counseling, raise questions about the general usefulness of sodium reduction....for hypertension in the general population."

Salt is an essential element in your diet and it is important that you get the highest quality, just as with any other nutrient. So let's talk a bit about what salt is best for you and what the food companies have done to make commercial salt a toxin rather than a nutrient.

The Tibetans are known for their longevity. Some credit their longevity to the consumption of apricot pits but that is a small part of the story. Researchers from Case Western Reserve University found the Tibetan diet to be totally incorrect

-- scientifically and politically – and yet they live a long, healthy life. The Phala nomads live on milk, butter, cheese, sheep, antelope, yak, and <u>practically no fruits or vegetables</u>. Their blood pressure averages are considerably lower than ours. <u>They consume a considerable amount of salt</u>.

There is a parallel between the stories of Demon Salt & Demon Cholesterol. The secretary at the front office often knows more about nutrition than her employer doctor. Doctors have been tragically misled on the cholesterol issue by the American Heart Association, universities, the government agencies and Congressional investigations, and the food industry. The same bad science & bad politics has plagued the issue of salt in the diet. The commercial food industry loves the anti-salt movement – it stimulates the sale of salt substitutes, which are more expensive.

All of our readers are aware that the refining of foods can reduce the food value of food and actually turn some foods into a toxic product. The best example of that is the homogenization of milk with its toxic xanthene oxidase levels. This could be a major factor in hypertension but, as far as I know, this theory has never been investigated. And it is possible that, if a correlation between salt & hypertension is ever conclusively proven, it is probably caused by the <u>massive consumption of commercial, refined salt</u>, not pure, unadulterated salt.

Let's give salt a fair shake:

- <u>Salt is an essential nutrient</u>, just like vitamin A, the fatty acids, and cholesterol.
- Vigorous restriction of salt in the diet may throw your other essential minerals into disarray and <u>induce</u> hypertension.
- Salt restriction in the summer months could lead to heat exhaustion, a severe mineral disturbance that causes fainting and sometimes a stroke or a heart attack in the susceptible elderly.
- The salt/hypertension research is conflicting and therefore has <u>proven nothing</u>.
- All professional, political and commercial organizations are urging you to restrict your salt intake – take this advice with a grain of salt.

Not all salts are created equal. Just like "Equal" is not sugar, "Morton's" is not salt or, at least, not one made for human consumption. <u>Morton's salt is an industrial product, made for the chemical industry, not your table</u>. Ninety percent of this industrial grade salt goes to the chemical industry and the rest to the grocery store.

'The only salt worthy of your consideration is sea salt from a clean sea bed. Salt mined from a Siberian salt mine is not sea salt, although it was from the sea 10,000 years ago. And all modern sea salts are not created equal. If you are using any of the "sea salts" but one, you are probably being short changed.

To be a sea salt worthy of your family, it must meet all three of the following criteria:

• Stick your finger in the container. You will note, if it is legitimate sea salt, it's a little soggy. When kept in cool storage, it doesn't dry out.

• The crystals, under magnification, are small and cubic.

If the salt is crystal white, it may be sea salt but it has been treated and fractionated to rid it of impurities and, at the same time, this rids it of essential minerals. If it is not light grey, it is not a nutritious salt. The moistness is due to the presence of magnesium salts. Morton is proud of its famous motto: "When it rains it pours." Their salt pours when it rains because it is <u>magnesium deficient</u> and it contains <u>sand</u>.

Ref: *Progress in Cardiovascular Diseases*, July / August, 1999

American Journal of Clinical Nutrition, Vol. 25, 1972
   Hypertension, Vol 18, 1991

American Journal of Clinical Nutrition, Vol 65, 1997
   Hypertension, Vol. 17, 1991

Journal of the American Medical Association, Vol. 267, 1992

American Journal of Medicine, Vol. 4, 1948

"When it rains it pours" applies to a lot of things. It has become a common household expression thanks to 100 years of ceaseless promotion by Morton. The industrial salt industry, meaning basically Morton, finagled the regulatory agency, CODEX, into slipping through a regulation that would allow the manufacturers to put up to two percent additives in their salt for human consumption. This included bleach, conditioners and anti-caking agents – <u>sand</u>.

So the old salts at Morton needed no further encouragement. They proceeded to extract the essential minerals, as well as the contaminants, from the salt and then sold the minerals back to the health industry and to industries requiring these minerals in their manufacturing process. The demineralized, nutrition-free, salt/sand combination goes to your dinner table – bon appetite!

There is nothing more important to your digestion than adequate whole salt. Salivary amylase, the primary digestive enzyme in the mouth, is activated by salt. Also in the mouth, salt activates the taste buds. Whereas, the "salt substitutes" (There IS no substitute, only other salts that are not sodium chloride, such as the popular potassium chloride.) only weakly stimulate the taste buds. So what does the deceived diner do? He adds <u>more</u> fake salt to his food to compensate and thereby gets as much sodium or more than he would with real salt.

Continuing down the digestive tract, salt stimulates the parietal cells of the stomach lining to generate hydrochloric acid, essential for proper digestion. Fake salt, i.e., potassium salt rather than sodium salt, blocks enzymatic pathways and thus interferes with hydrochloric acid production. That indigestion you have may not be caused by <u>too much</u> acid but by <u>too little</u> – the symptoms are the same for either condition – and KCL (potassium chloride) may be the culprit.

Nutritional scientists have worried about <u>too much</u> salt in the diet and, until recently, have ignored the place of <u>too little</u> salt in the panoply of human disease. But, <u>as we have shown you from the medical literature itself</u>, a low salt diet may have serious consequences. This brings us to the serious problem of vegetarians who eat a low-salt diet.

Vegetarians tend to be extremists in their own misguided way. They will not pay any attention to the scientific literature unless it agrees with their own opinions. I have given up on them but this will be of interest to you because you may have a child, or grandchild, who seems to be meandering down the Turnip Trail. Remember, in your attempt to save this child, you will have to fight the bear huggers, asp kissers and carrot suckers every step of the way. It's a daunting task – and we are losing.

Being puritanical in nature, vegetarians like to deny themselves things that are fun and/or taste good. Salt is the great enhancer of flavor but the vegetarians (secretly) think it is sugar. (They absolutely can not resist sugar – I'll explain that in a minute.) Go to any farm and the grazing animals will tell you that salt is vital to them and to their grazing cousins, homo sapio-vegetarious. These herbivores will tell you that salt is the single element required for the proper breakdown of plant carbohydrate into usable food. <u>That's why they hang around</u> <u>the salt lick</u>. The farmer and the cows know salt is vital to the health of <u>all</u> vegetarian mammals but they've also given up on the human grass eaters.

If they won't eat Bambi or Flipper, they should at least eat salt. Even properly-grown vegetables and fruits are practically salt-free. Domestically-grown plants come even closer to zero in salt content. That's why salt sprinkled on carrots and cantaloupe causes the flavor to literally burst forth. It does the same for chicken. A vegetarian can graze constantly (and many do) in an attempt to meet his salt needs, but he will never succeed. That's why they die young and go to vegetarian heaven where every animal is an inedible pet and they can have all the salt and ice cream they want. They can wear their "Smokey the Bear" medal with pride. They kept the faith and did their best.

I promised to tell you about the sugar addiction of vegetarians. Glycosides in grains are not digested without the presence of salt. If the vegan does not supplement his third-world diet with salt, the body is denied these natural sugars, they develop a glycoside deficiency and with it comes an insatiable craving for ice cream, cake, pie, doughnuts, candy, and anything -- sweet or salted -- sold at the neighborhood movie theatre.

If you restrict your salt intake, you are also risking a magnesium deficiency. The elderly are more prone to develop magnesium deficiency. A lack of magnesium appears to be related to impotence and senility. Many soils, especially in the mid-west, are magnesium- deficient and if the soil is deficient, the plants will be deficient. Studies have shown that particular areas with low magnesium in the soil have higher rates of heart disease.

The word has gotten out that "French sea salt" is the way to go. But just because the label says "French salt" doesn't mean it is any better than Morton's salt. Opportunists have gotten on the salt wagon and are spraying their clot-free and nutrition-free French salt all over the world.

The world authority on salt is Dr. Jacques de Langre. For an excellent lesson in salt science and salt lore, read on:

"Cold, active, northern seas, because of upwelling and other marine and climactic conditions, offer the advantages of a rich mix of minerals....Winds not only dry more than sun alone, but 'load' the salt flats and stack with additional trace elements, mainly iodine salts. These additional nutrients are carried as spray from the crests of waves...."

"The method used for gathering salt from natural flats and effectively separating it from the hard soil is crucial to the production of health-giving salt. There must be some constant eddying movement in the brine – a kinetic crystallization – over and through the clay flats....In order to ionize and harmonize the trace elements by the clay's filtering action, the final hand-raking of the moist crystals is done by artisans with such a skillful, light touch that almost no particles of clay appear in the finished natural product.

"In the case of 'Flower of the Ocean' salt, an almost white Celtic salt which is harvested traditionally and is rare because it crystallizes naturally on top of the water only on the hottest days of the harvest, contains no clay particles at all and yields tiny white crystals. The gathering is done delicately from the top layer of the brine and thus no clay is ever trapped in the final, smaller crystal structure.

"Both methods just described are still followed by a dedicated group of professional natural salt farmers in Europe who perpetuate the traditional skills down through generations from antiquity. When harvested in these ways, both of these natural sea salts are highly beneficial to anyone's health as they possess therapeutic qualities that are capable of restoring balance, even in long-standing chronic afflictions."

Action to take:

If you have a normal blood pressure, or a slight elevation that remains stable, salt restriction is not warranted. If you have enlargement of the left side of the heart (left ventricular hypertrophy), salt restriction will be necessary and may improve the heart condition whether you have hypertension or not. This is paradoxical and has not been explained.

Use the best salt available and that is Celtic sea salt. The address for this vital nutrient is:

> The Grain & Salt Society
> 273 Fairway Dr.
> Ashville, NC 28805

Ref:

American Journal of Hypertension, 2001; 14:397-404

Progress in Cardiovascular Diseases, July / August, 1999

American Journal of Clinical Nutrition, Vol. 25, 1972

Hypertension, Vol. 18, 1991

American Journal of Clinical Nutrition, Vol 65, 1997

Hypertension, Vol. 17, 1991

Journal of the American Medical Association, Vol. 267, 1992

American Journal of Medicine, Vol. 4, 1948

Hypertension, Vol. 30:150

Hypertension, 2000; Vol 36,171

####

About Doctor William Campbell Douglass II

Dr. Douglass reveals medical truths, and deceptions, often at risk of being labeled heretical. He is consumed by a passion for living a long healthy life, and wants his readers to share that passion. Their health and well-being comes first. He is anti-dogmatic, and unwavering in his dedication to improve the quality of life of his readers. He has been called "the conscience of modern medicine," a "medical maverick," and has been voted "Doctor of the Year" by the National Health Federation. His medical experiences are far reaching-from battling malaria in Central America - to fighting deadly epidemics at his own health clinic in Africa - to flying with U.S. Navy crews as a flight surgeon - to working for 10 years in emergency medicine here in the States. These learning experiences, not to mention his keen storytelling ability and wit, make Dr. Douglass' newsletters (Daily Dose and Real Health) and books uniquely interesting and fun to read. He shares his no-frills, no-bull approach to health care, often amazing his readers by telling them to ignore many widely-hyped good-health practices (like staying away from red meat, avoiding coffee, and eating like a bird), and start living again by eating REAL food, taking some inexpensive supplements, and doing the pleasurable things that make life livable. Readers get all this, plus they learn how to burn fat, prevent cancer, boost libido, and so much more. And, Dr. Douglass is not afraid to challenge the latest studies that come out, and share the real story with his readers. Dr. William C. Douglass has led a colorful, rebellious, and crusading life. Not many physicians would dare put their professional reputations on the line as many times as this courageous healer has. A vocal opponent of "business-as-usual" medicine, Dr. Douglass has championed patients' rights and physician commitment to wellness throughout his career. This dedicated physician has repeatedly gone far beyond the call of duty in his work to spread the truth about alternative therapies. For a full year, he endured economic and physical hardship to work with physicians at the Pasteur Institute in St. Petersburg, Russia, where advanced research on photoluminescence was being conducted. Dr. Douglass comes from a distinguished family of physicians. He is the fourth generation Douglass to practice medicine, and his son is also a physician. Dr. Douglass graduated from the University of Rochester, the Miami School of Medicine, and the Naval School of Aviation and Space Medicine.

You want to protect those you love from the health dangers the authorities aren't telling you about, and learn the incredible cures that they've scorned and ignored?
Subscribe to the free Daily Dose updates "...the straight scoop about health, medicine, and politics." by sending an e-mail to real_sub@agoramail.net with the word "subscribe" in the subject line.

Dr. William Campbell Douglass'
Real Health:

Had Enough?

Enough turkey burgers and sprouts?

Enough forcing gallons of water down your throat?

Enough exercising until you can barely breathe?

Before you give up everything just because "everyone" says it's healthy...

Learn the facts from Dr. William Campbell Douglass, medicine's most acclaimed myth-buster. In every issue of Dr. Douglass' Real Health newsletter, you'll learn shocking truths about "junk medicine" and how to stay healthy while eating eggs, meat and other foods you love.

With the tips you'll receive from Real Health, you'll see your doctor less, spend a lot less money and be happier and healthier while you're at it. The road to Real Health is actually easier, cheaper and more pleasant than you dared to dream.

Subscribe to Real Health today by calling 1-800-981-7162 or visit the Real Health web site at www.realhealthnews.com.
Use promotional code : DRHBDZZZ

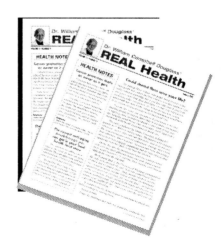

If you knew of a procedure that could save thousands, maybe millions, of people dying from AIDS, cancer, and other dreaded killers....

Would you cover it up?

It's unthinkable that what could be the best solution ever to stopping the world's killer diseases is being ignored, scorned, and rejected. But that is exactly what's happening right now.

The procedure is called "photoluminescence". It's a thoroughly tested, proven therapy that uses the healing power of the light to perform almost miraculous cures.

This remarkable treatment works its incredible cures by stimulating the body's own immune responses. That's why it cures so many ailments--and why it's been especially effective against AIDS! Yet, 50 years ago, it virtually disappeared from the halls of medicine.

Why has this incredible cure been ignored by the medical authorities of this country? You'll find the shocking answer here in the pages of this new edition of Into the Light. Now available with the blood irradiation Instrument Diagram and a complete set of instructions for building your own "Treatment Device". Also includes details on how to use this unique medical instrument.

Into the Light

*Into
the
Light*

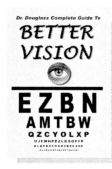

Dr. Douglass' Complete Guide to Better Vision

A report about eyesight and what can be done to improve it naturally. But I've also included information about how the eye works, brief descriptions of various common eye conditions, traditional remedies to eye problems, and a few simple suggestions that may help you maintain your eyesight for years to come.
-William Campbell Douglass II, MD

The Hypertension Report.
Say Good Bye to High Blood Pressure.

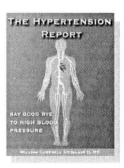

An estimated 50 million Americans have high blood pressure. Often called the "silent killer" because it may not cause symptoms until the patient has suffered serious damage to the arterial system. Diet, exercise, potassium supplements chelation therapy and practically anything but drugs is the way to go and alternatives are discussed in this report.

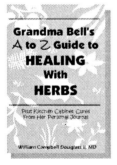

Grandma Bell's A To Z Guide To Healing With Herbs.

This book is all about - coming home. What I once believed to be old wives' tales - stories long destroyed by the new world of science - actually proved to be the best treatment for many of the common ailments you and I suffer through. So I put a few of them together in this book with the sincere hope that Grandma Bell's wisdom will help you recover your common sense, and take responsibility for your own health. -William Campbell Douglass II, MD

Prostate Problems:
Safe, Simple, Effective Relief for Men over 50.

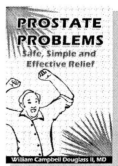

Don't be frightened into surgery or drugs you may not need. First, get the facts about prostate problems... know all your options, so you can make the best decisions. This fully documented report explains the dangers of conventional treatments, and gives you alternatives that could save you more than just money!

Color me Healthy
The Healing Powers of Colors

"He's crazy!"
"He's got to be a quack!"
"Who gave this guy his medical license?"
"He's a nut case!"

In case you're wondering, those are the reactions you'll probably get if you show your doctor this report. I know the idea of healing many common ailments simply by exposing them to colored light sounds far-fetched, but when you see the evidence, you'll agree that color is truly an amazing medical breakthrough.

When I first heard the stories,
I reacted much the same way.
But the evidence so
convinced me, that I had to
try color therapy in my practice.
My results were truly amazing.

-William Campbell Douglass II, MD

Order your complete set of Roscolene filters (choice of 3 sizes) to be used with the "Color Me Healthy" therapy. The eleven Roscolene filters are # 809, 810, 818, 826, 828, 832, 859, 861, 866, 871, and 877. The filters come with protective separator sheets between each filter. The color names and the Roscolene filter(s) used to produce that particular color, are printed on a card included with the filters and a set of instructions on how to fit them to a lamp.

Rhino Publishing
www.rhinopublish.com

What Is Going on Here?

Peroxides are supposed to be bad for you. Free radicals and all that. But now we hear that hydrogen peroxide is good for us. Hydrogen peroxide will put extra oxygen in your blood. There's no doubt about that. Hydrogen peroxide costs pennies. So if you can get oxygen into the blood cheaply and safely, maybe cancer (which doesn't like oxygen), emphysema, AIDS, and many other terrible diseases can be treated effectively. Intravenous hydrogen peroxide rapidly relieves allergic reactions, influenza symptoms, and acute viral infections.

No one expects to live forever. But we would all like to have a George Burns finish. The prospect of finishing life in a nursing home after abandoning your tricycle in the mobile home park is not appealing. Then comes the loss of control of vital functions the ultimate humiliation. Is life supposed to be from tricycle to tricycle and diaper to diaper? You come into this world crying, but do you have to leave crying? I don't believe you do. And you won't either after you see the evidence. Sounds too good to be true, doesn't it? Read on and decide for yourself.

-William Campbell Douglass II, MD

Rhino Publishing S.A.
www.rhinopublish.com

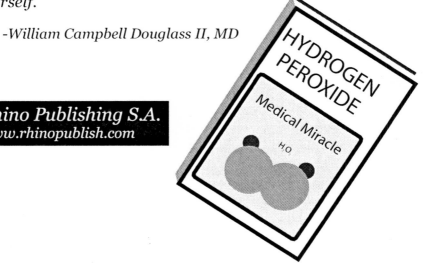

Don't drink your milk!

If you knew what we know about milk... BLEECHT! All that pasteurization, homogenization and processing is not only cooking all the nutrients right out of your favorite drink. It's also adding toxic levels of vitamin D.

This fascinating book tells the whole story about milk. How it once was nature's perfect food...how "raw," unprocessed milk can heal and boost your immune system ... why you can't buy it legally in this country anymore, and what we could do to change that.

Dr. "Douglass traveled all over the world, tasting all kinds of milk from all kinds of cows, poring over dusty research books in ancient libraries far from home, to write this light-hearted but scientifically sound book.

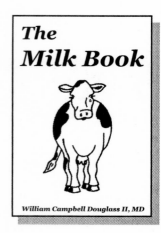

The
Milk Book

William Campbell Douglass II, MD

Rhino Publishing, S.A.
www.rhinopublish.com

Eat Your Cholesterol!

Eat Meat, Drink Milk, Spread The Butter- And Live Longer!
How to Live off the Fat of the Land and Feel Great.

Americans are being saturated with anti-cholesterol propaganda. If you watch very much television, you're probably one of the millions of Americans who now has a terminal case of cholesterol phobia. The propaganda is relentless and is often designed to produce fear and loathing of this worst of all food contaminants. You never hear the food propagandists bragging about their product being fluoride-free or aluminum-free, two of our truly serious food-additive problems. But cholesterol, an essential nutrient, not proven to be harmful in any quantity, is constantly pilloried as a menace to your health. If you don't use corn oil, Fleischmann's margarine, and Egg Beaters, you're going straight to atherosclerosis hell with stroke, heart attack, and premature aging -- and so are your kids. Never feel guilty about what you eat again! Dr. Douglass shows you why red meat, eggs, and dairy products aren't the dietary demons we're told they are. But beware: This scientifically sound report goes against all the "common wisdom" about the foods you should eat. Read with an open mind.

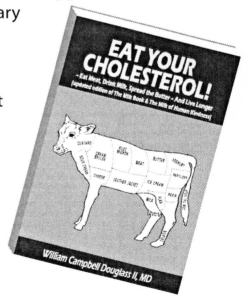

Rhino Publishing, S.A.
www.rhinopublish.com

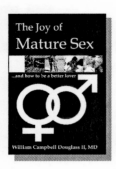

The Joy of Mature Sex
and How to Be a Better Lover

Humans are very confused about what makes good sex. But I believe humans have more to offer each other than this total licentiousness common among animals. We're talking about mature sex. The kind of sex that made this country great.

Stop Aging or Slow the Process
How Exercise With Oxygen Therapy
(EWOT) Can Help

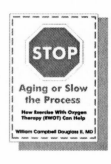

EWOT (pronounced ee-watt) stands for Exercise With Oxygen Therapy. This method of prolonging your life is so simple and you can do it at home at a minimal cost. When your cells don't get enough oxygen, they degenerate and die and so you degenerate and die. It's as simple as that.

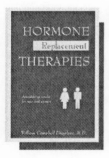

Hormone Replacement Therapies:
Astonishing Results For Men And Women

It is accurate to say that when the endocrine glands start to fail, you start to die. We are facing a sea change in longevity and health in the elderly. Now, with the proper supplemental hormones, we can slow the aging process and, in many cases, reverse some of the signs and symptoms of aging.

Add 10 Years to Your Life
With some "best of" Dr. Douglass' writings.

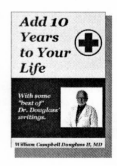

To add ten years to your life, you need to have the right attitude about health and an understanding of the health industry and what it's feeding you. Following the established line on many health issues could make you very sick or worse! Achieve dynamic health with this collection of some of the "best of" Dr. Douglass' newsletters.

How did AIDS become one of the Greatest Biological Disasters in the History of Mankind?

GET THE FACTS

AIDS and BIOLOGICAL WARFARE covers the history of plagues from the past to today's global confrontation with AIDS, the Prince of Plagues. Completely documented *AIDS and BIOLOGICAL WARFARE* helps you make your own decisions about how to survive in a world ravaged by this horrible plague.

You will learn that AIDS is not a naturally occuring disease process as you have been led to believe, but a man-made biological nightmare that has been unleashed and is now threatening the very existence of human life on the planet.

There is a smokescreen of misinformation clouding the AIDS issue. Now, for the first time, learn the truth about the nature of the crisis our planet faces: its origin -- how AIDS is really transmited and alternatives for treatment. Find out what they are not telling you about AIDS and Biological Warfare, and how to protect yourself and your loved ones. AIDS is a serious problem worldwide, but it is no longer the major threat. You need to know the whole story. To protect yourself, you must know the truth about biological warfare.

Rhino Publishing S.A.
www.rhinopublish.com

PAINFUL DILEMMA

Are we fighting the wrong war?

We are spending millions on the war against drugs while we
should be fighting the war against pain with those drugs!

As you will read in this book, the war on drugs was lost a long time ago and,
when it comes to the war against pain, pain is winning! An article in USA Today
(11/20/02) reveals that dying patients are not getting relief from pain. It seems
the doctors are torn between fear of the government, certainly justified, and a
clinging to old and out dated ideas about pain, which is NOT justified.

A group called Last Acts, a coalition of health-care groups, has released a very
discouraging study of all 50 states that nearly half of the 1.6 million Americans
living in nursing homes suffer from untreated pain. They said that life was being
extended but it amounted to little more than "extended pain and suffering."

This book offers insight into the history of pain treatment and the current failed
philosophies of contemporary medicine. Plus it describes some of today's most
advanced treatments for alleviating certain kinds of pain. This book is not another
"self-help" book touting home remedies; rather, Painful Dilemma: Patients in
Pain -- People in Prison, takes a hard look at where we've gone wrong and what
we (you) can do to help a loved one who is living with chronic pain.

The second half of this book is a must read if you value your freedom. We now
have the ridiculous and tragic situation of people
in pain living in a government-created hell by
restriction of narcotics and people in prison for
trying to bring pain relief by the selling of
narcotics to the suffering. The end result of the
"war on drugs" has been to create the greatest
and most destructive cartel in history, so great,
in fact, that the drug Mafia now controls most
of the world economy.

Rhino Publishing S.A.
www.rhinopublish.com

Live the Adventure!

Why would anyone in their right mind put everything they own in storage and move to Russia, of all places?! But when maverick physician Bill Douglass left a profitable medical practice in a peaceful mountaintop town to pursue "pure medical truth".... none of us who know him well was really surprised.

After All, anyone who's braved the outermost reaches of darkest Africa, the mean streets of Johannesburg and New York, and even a trip to Washington to testify before the Senate, wouldn't bat and eye at ducking behind the Iron Curtain for a little medical reconnaissance!

Enjoy this imaginative, funny, dedicated man's tales of wonder and woe as he treks through a year in St. Petersburg, working on a cure for the world's killer diseases. We promise --

YOU WON'T BE BORED!

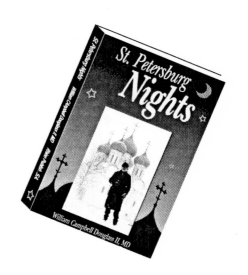

Rhino Publishing S.A.
www.rhinopublish.com

THE SMOKER'S PARADOX
THE HEALTH BENEFITS OF TOBACCO!

The benefits of smoking tobacco have been common knowledge for centuries. From sharpening mental acuity to maintaining optimal weight, the relatively small risks of smoking have always been outweighed by the substantial improvement to mental and physical health. Hysterical attacks on tobacco notwithstanding, smokers always weigh the good against the bad and puff away or quit according to their personal preferences. Now the same anti-tobacco enterprise that has spent billions demonizing the pleasure of smoking is providing additional reasons to smoke. Alzheimer's, Parkinson's, Tourette's Syndrome, even schizophrenia and cocaine addiction are disorders that are alleviated by tobacco. Add in the still inconclusive indication that tobacco helps to prevent colon and prostate cancer and the endorsement for smoking tobacco by the medical establishment is good news for smokers and non-smokers alike. Of course the revelation that tobacco is good for you is ruined by the pharmaceutical industry's plan to substitute the natural and relatively inexpensive tobacco plant with their overpriced and ineffective nicotine substitutions. Still, when all is said and done, the positive revelations regarding tobacco are very good reasons indeed to keep lighting those cigars - but only 4 a day!

THE SMOKER'S
PARADOX
William Campbell Douglass II, MD

The health
benefits of
tobacco

Rhino Publishing, S.A
www.rhinopublish.com

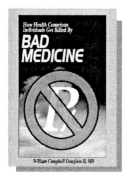

Bad Medicine
How Individuals Get Killed By Bad Medicine.

Do you really need that new prescription or that overnight stay in the hospital? In this report, Dr. Douglass reveals the common medical practices and misconceptions endangering your health. Best of all, he tells you the pointed (but very revealing!) questions your doctor prays you never ask. Interesting medical facts about popular remedies are revealed.

Dangerous Legal Drugs
The Poisons in Your Medicine Chest.

If you knew what we know about the most popular prescription and over-the-counter drugs, you'd be sick. That's why Dr. Douglass wrote this shocking report about the poisons in your medicine chest. He gives you the low-down on different categories of drugs. Everything from painkillers and cold remedies to tranquilizers and powerful cancer drugs.

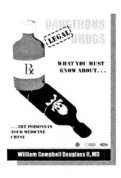

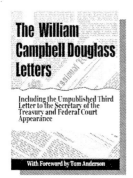

The William Campbell Douglass Letters.
Expose of Government Machinations
(Vietnam War).

THE WILLIAM CAMPBELL DOUGLASS LETTERS. Dr. Douglass' Defense in 1968 Tax Case and Expose of Government Machinations during the Vietnam War.

The Eagle's Feather. A Novel of
International Political Intrigue.

Although The Eagle's Feather is a work of fiction set in the 1970's, it is built, as with most fiction, on a framework of plausibility and background information. This is a fiction book that could not have been written were it not for various ominous aspects, which pose a clear and present danger to the security of the United States.

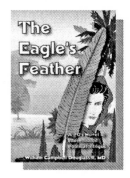

Rhino Publishing

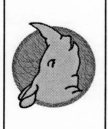

ORDER FORM

PURCHASER INFORMATION

Purchaser's Name (Please Print): _____

Shipping Address (Do not use a P.O. Box): _____

City: _____ State/Prov.: _____ Country: _____

Zip/Postal Code: _____ Telephone No.: _____ Fax No.: _____

E-Mail Address (if interested in receiving free e-Books when available): _____

CREDIT CARD INFO (CIRCLE ONE):

MASTERCARD, VISA, AMERICAN EXPRESS, DISCOVER, JCB, DINER'S CLUB, CARTE BLANCHE.

Charge my Card -> Number #: _____ Exp.: _____

*Security Code: _____ * Required for all MasterCard, Visa and American Express purchases. For your security, we require that you enter your card's verification number. The verification number is also called a CCV number. This code is the 3 digits farthest right in the signature field on the back of your VISA/MC, or the 4 digits to the right on the front of your American Express card. Your credit card statement will show **a different name than Rhino Publishing** as the vendor.

WE DO NOT share your private information, we use 3rd party credit card processing service to process your order only.

ADDITIONAL INFORMATION

If your shipping address is not the same as your credit card billing address, please indicate your card billing address here.

_____   _____
Name on the card   Type of card:

Billing Address: _____

City: _____ State/Prov.: _____ Zip/Postal Code: _____

Fax a copy of this order to:
RHINO PUBLISHING, S.A.
1-888-317-6767 or International #: + 416-352-5126

To order by mail, send your payment by first class mail only to the following address. Please include a copy of this order form. Make your check or bank drafts (NO postal money order) payable to RHINO PUBLISHING, S.A. and mail to:

Rhino Publishing, S.A.
Attention: PTY 5048
P.O. Box 025724
Miami, FL.
USA 33102

Digital E-books also available online: www.rhinopublish.com

Rhino Publishing

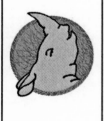

ORDER FORM

Purchaser's Name (Please Print): _____

I would like to order the following paperback book of Dr. Douglass (Alternative Medicine Books):

___	X	9962-636-04-3	Add 10 Years to Your Life. With some "best of" Dr. Douglass writings.	$13.99 $ ___
___	X	9962-636-07-8	AIDS and Biological Warfare. What They Are Not Telling You!	$17.99 $ ___
___	X	9962-636-09-4	Bad Medicine. How Individuals Get Killed By Bad Medicine.	$11.99 $ ___
___	X	9962-636-10-8	Color Me Healthy. The Healing Power of Colors.	$11.99 $ ___
___	X	9962-636 -XX-X	Color Filters for Color Me Healthy. 11 Basic Roscolene Filters for Lamps.	$21.89 $ ___
___	X	9962-636-15-9	Dangerous Legal Drugs. The Poisons in Your Medicine Chest.	$13.99 $ ___
___	X	9962-636-18-3	Dr. Douglass' Complete Guide to Better Vision. Improve eyesight naturally.	$11.99 $ ___
___	X	9962-636-19-1	Eat Your Cholesterol! How to Live off the Fat of the Land and Feel Great.	$11.99 $ ___
___	X	9962-636-12-4	Grandma Bell's A To Z Guide To Healing. Her Kitchen Cabinet Cures.	$14.99 $ ___
___	X	9962-636-22-1	Hormone Replacement Therapies. Astonishing Results For Men & Women	$11.99 $ ___
___	X	9962-636-25-6	Hydrogen Peroxide: One of the Most Underused Medical Miracle.	$15.99 $ ___
___	X	9962-636-27-2	Into the Light. New Edition with Blood Irradiation Instrument Instructions.	$19.99 $ ___
___	X	9962-636-54-X	Milk Book. The Classic on the Nutrition of Milk and How to Benefit from it.	$17.99 $ ___

___	X	9962-636-00-0	Painful Dilemma - Patients in Pain - People in Prison.	$17.99	$ ___
___	X	9962-636-32-9	Prostate Problems. Safe, Simple, Effective Relief for Men over 50.	$11.99	$ ___
___	X	9962-636-34-5	St. Petersburg Nights. Enlightening Story of Life and Science in Russia.	$17.99	$ ___
___	X	9962-636-37-X	Stop Aging or Slow the Process. Exercise With Oxygen Therapy Can Help.	$11.99	$ ___
___	X	9962-636-60-4	The Hypertension Report. Say Good Bye to High Blood Pressure.	$11.99	$ ___
___	X	9962-636-48-5	The Joy of Mature Sex and How to Be a Better Lover...	$13.99	$ ___
___	X	9962-636-43-4	The Smoker's Paradox: Health Benefits of Tobacco.	$14.99	$ ___

Political Books:

___	X	9962-636-40-X	The Eagle's Feather. A 70's Novel of International Political Intrigue.	$15.99	$ ___
___	X	9962-636-46-9	The W. C. D. Letters. Expose of Government Machinations (Vietnam War).	$11.99	$ ___

SUB-TOTAL: $ ___

ADD $5.00 HANDLING FOR YOUR ORDER: $ 5.00 $ 5.00

___ X ADD $2.50 SHIPPING FOR EACH ITEM ON ORDER: $ 2.50 $ ___

NOTE THAT THE MINIMUM SHIPPING AND HANDLING IS $7.50 FOR 1 BOOK ($5.00 + $2.50)
For order shipped outside the US, add $5.00 per item

___ X ADD $5.00 S. & H. OR EACH ITEM ON ORDER (INTERNATIONAL ORDERS ONLY) $ 5.00 $ ___

Allow up to 21 days for delivery (we will call you about back orders if any)

TOTAL: $ ___

Fax a copy of this order to: 1-888-317-6767 or Int'l + 416-352-5126
or mail to: Rhino Publishing, S.A. Attention: PTY 5048 P.O. Box 025724, Miami, FL., 33102 USA
Digital E-books also available online: www.rhinopublish.com

Printed in the United States
1503500001B/11